28 SECRETS ABOUT HAIR GROWTH

Marcia Savage

How To Grow Longer, Thicker Hair Fast

Disclaimer and/or Legal Notices

Your Free Gift

As a way of saying thanks for your purchase, I'm offering a free guide that's exclusive to my readers.

In this guide, you will learn how to turn any messy room in into a nice, clean, and tidy room, cleaning in only 3 hours. Your home will stay clean every day and you will never have to worry about unexpected guests walking into a dirty house again. You can download this free report by going here.

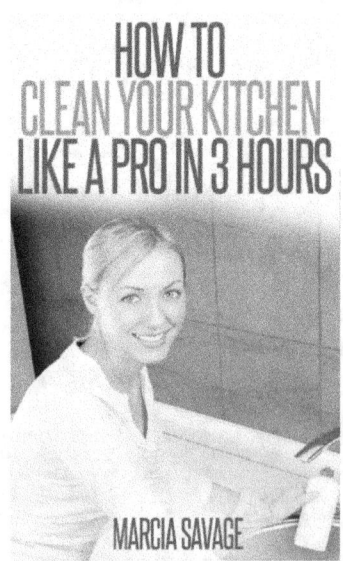

http://forms.aweber.com/form/76/315836976.htm

Table Of Contents

Vitamin-Mineral Supplement

Fresh Ginger Root

Do Not Brush Your Hair When Wet

Wash Your Hair

Use Natural Hair Care Products

Use Products To Moisturize Your Hair

Conditioning Your Hair

Trim Your Hair Regularly

Protect Your Hair

Protect Your Hair at Bedtime

Massaging Your Scalp Daily

Use Prenatal Supplements

Grape Seed Oil

Cactus Leaves

Garlic, Onions, an Cinnamon Sticks

Birth Control Pills and Your Shampoo

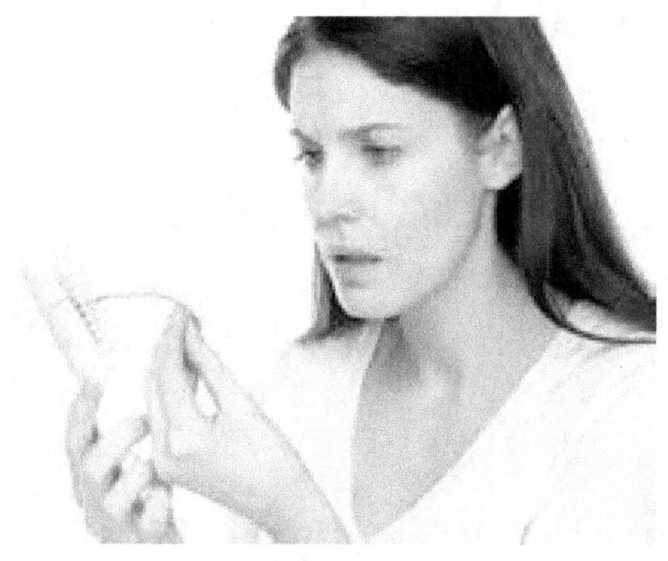

Hair loss can be a depressing experience for most people. Some people choose to ignore it, hoping their hair will grow back, while others spend their hard earned money trying every product on the market. Let me tell you a little secret. 'You may have the cure to hair loss right in your home.' Do I have your attention now?

Hello! My name is Marcia Savage and just like most 30+ year old women, I have experienced hair loss, but I have an ace in the hole because my mother, grandmother and their parents all had the same problem. But they found natural home solutions that not only cured their hair loss, but made their stronger, healthier, and longer, fast. Do you want to cure hair loss? Do you want longer, fuller, and healthier hair in the next 30 days? Well, buckle your seat belt because we are about to go on one hell of a drive. Are you ready? Let's get started.

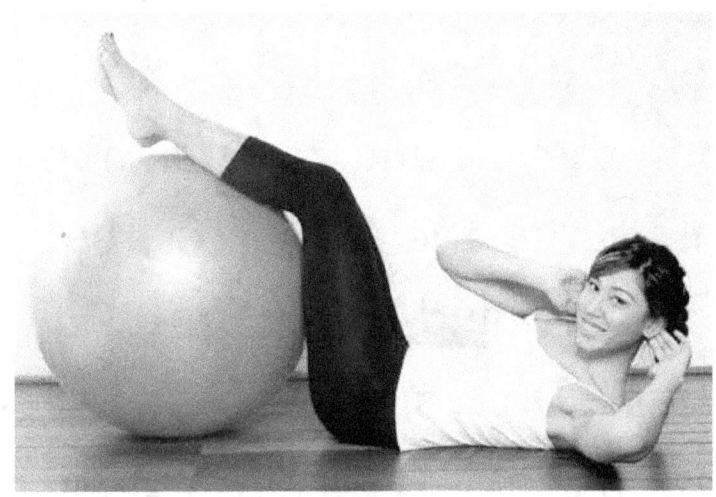

The first step to healthy hair is a healthy body. To prove what I'm saying is true, have you ever seen a healthy person whose hair falls out? You should try to do some type of exercise 3 to 4 times a week. I know it's a pain in the butt but if you want to grow hair back fast, exercise.

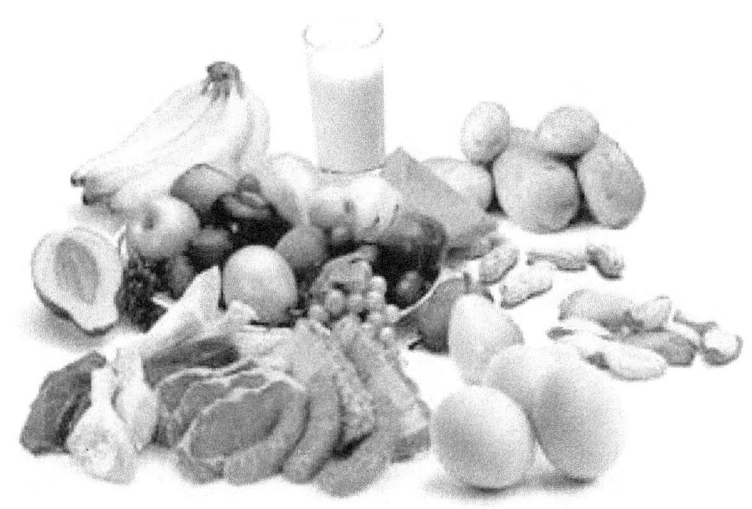

A healthy diet of meat and vegetables will not only cut fat, but will recover hair loss. If you want to regrow your hair fast, find a simple diet of fish, meat, fruit, and vegetables and stick with it. Believe me, my friend, this really works.

Have Protein With Every Meal

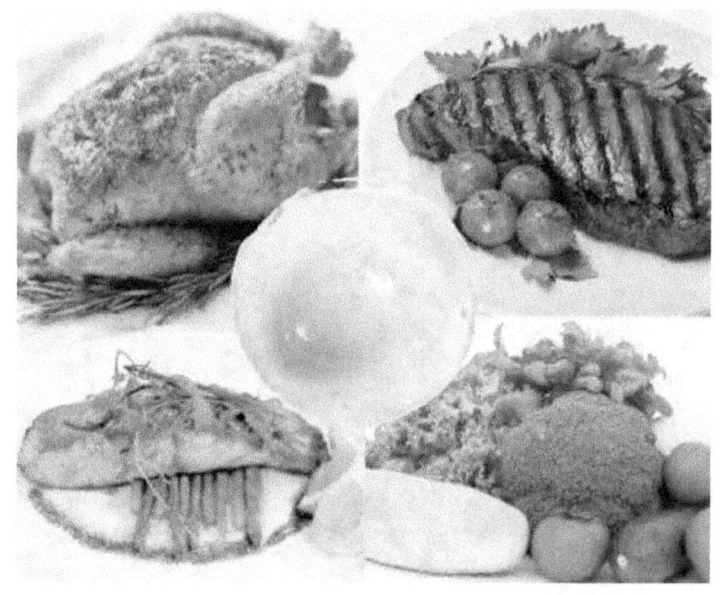

Protein not only builds muscle mass, but it builds hair and restores hair loss. You should consume some type of protein every meal. But lean protein like fish, steak, chicken breast, pork, and eggs are healthier proteins that are also good for your body.

Eat Shrimp

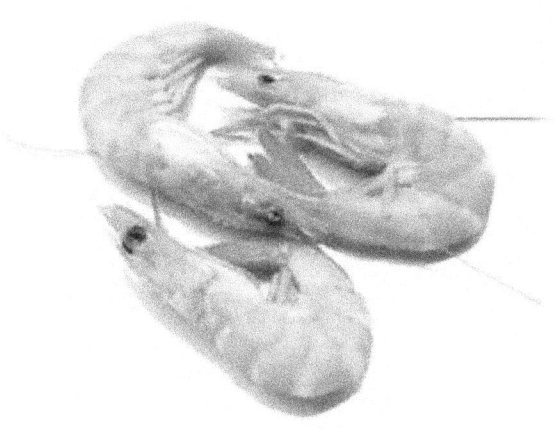

If you are a shrimp lover, I have good news. Shrimp is loaded with protein, which can help your hair and nails grow faster. They also contain, zinc, and vitamin B12, which is good hair nourishment and prevent hair loss. So, if you love it, enjoy it, because shrimp can also help you live longer.

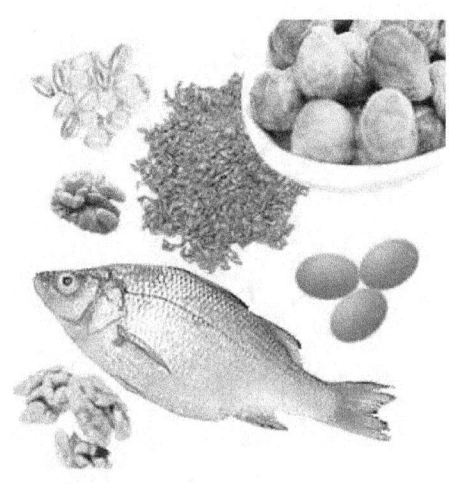

If you wondering about what vitamins can help when it comes to hair growth, then you should consume foods full of zinc and essential fatty acids. The reason why is because these substance can prevent dry scalp and dandruff. Eating foods that contain lots of zinc and fatty acids will make your hair fuller and healthier, and will make it grow.

This may sound simple but it's true, every man and woman should drink one gallon of water or more every day. Water not only promotes good health, but also promotes hair growth.

Start your day off with one glass of water and follow up with one glass of water every 2 hours throughout the day.

Hair Mask Treatment One

You'll need:

3 Tbsp. of Coconut Oil

2 Tbsp. of Honey

Step One: Make a paste by mixing the solution together.

Step Two: Warm the honey and coconut oil in microwave and put it on your hair as mask.

Step Three: Cover your head with shower cap and wash after 30 minutes.

Hair Mask Treatment Two

You'll need:

½ of an Avocado

2 Tbsp. Honey

Step One: Smash up the avocado, add honey, and mix to paste.

Step Two: Warm the avocado and honey in the microwave and put on your hair as mask.

Step Three: Cover your hair with a shower cap and wash after 30 minutes.

Honey and Aloe Vera

You'll need:

Aloe Vera Plant

1 Tbsp. Honey

Step One: Cut off a small branch of Aloe Vera, and scrape off its gel.

Step Two: Mix the gel thoroughly in a bowl with one tablespoon of honey, and apply it to the scalp.

Step Three: Leave it on for 20 minutes, and rinse away with harm water.

Lemon Juice and Onion

Did you know lemon juice and onion contain essential nutrients that stimulate your hair follicles? For a simple natural recipe, try the following:

Step One: Mix equal proportions of onion and lemon juice in a bowl.

Step Two: Use this solution when you massage your scalp, and work it into your hair.

Step Three: Leave the solution on for 30 minutes and rinse it with warm water.

Boiling Celery Leaves and Lemon Juice

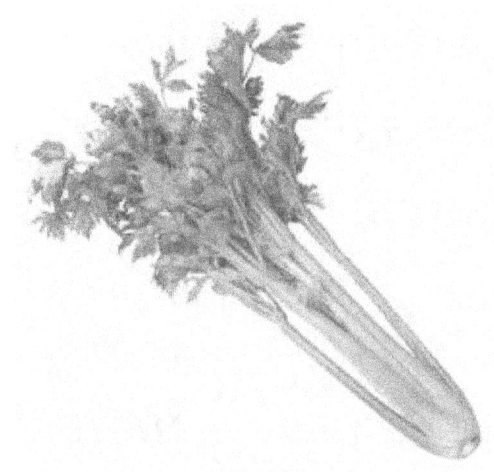

Rubbing boiled celery leaves and lemon juice on your scalp will make your hair grow long fast because this solution contains essential nutrients that can promote healthy hair grow. Apply this mixture after you shampoo your hair for results you can see in just a matter of weeks.

Minced Onion and Shampoo

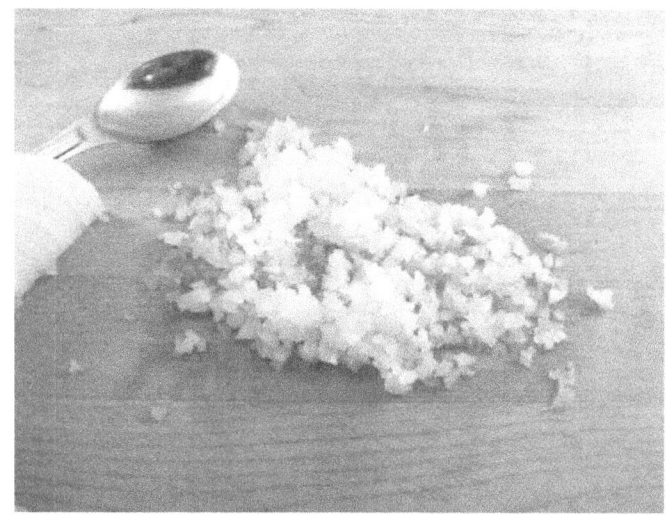

Adding minced onions to your shampoo will make your hair grow faster. Mince your onions into small pieces and add it into the bottle of shampoo, and let it stand for 60 minutes, before washing your hair. Not only will it make your hair grow, it will also make your hair shine more.

Biotin Vitamins

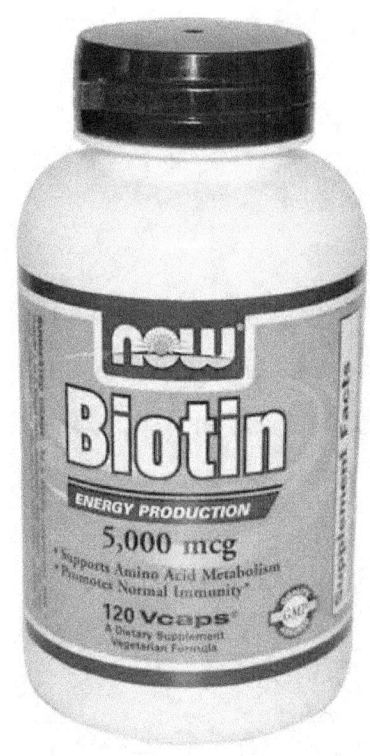

If you want to grow hair faster, take Biotin vitamins every day. I take one 5000 mg Biotin vitamin a day, every morning with one glass of water. I bought it at Rid Aid drug store but you can find it at any local drug store.

Vitamin-Mineral Supplement

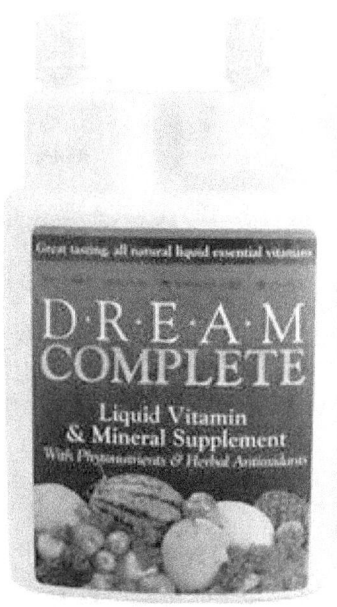

The best way to be sure you are getting the right vitamins and minerals is to take a supplement. We need the right vitamins and mineral for proper hair growth. Make sure you are buying 'Complete Vitamins', because they will enhance the growth of your hair. You can find it at any local drug store.

Fresh Ginger Root

If you are trying to treat bald spots and thinning hair, fresh ginger roots are the answer. This hair loss cure is over 5000 years old and said to be used by the Egyptian pharaohs.

Step One: Peel the skin off the ginger root, removing the hard skin until you expose the flesh of the soft skin.

Step Two: Cut the skin into small pieces so it easy to blend.

Step Three: Drop all the pieces into the blender, add three tablespoons of water, and continue adding water until you turn the mixture into a juice.

Do not ever comb or brush your hair when it is wet. Because combing or brushing wet hair will tear it out by the roots. You should blow dry your hair before you comb or brush it.

If you are using a comb, use a wide tooth plastic comb and always begin combing and brushing your hair on the ends working inward. This will loosen entangled hair from the ends.

Wash Your Hair

Shampoo your hair 3 times a week. Dirt and dust clogs the scalp and will prevent hair growth. I try to wash my hair every other day. You should not wash your hair every day because the shampoo will remove the oils your scalp produces so it will not be able to grow.

Use Natural Hair Care Products

Most hair care products are loaded with synthetic substances that can harm your hair. It would be wise to stay away from them. You should look for products that are made out of natural substances.

These types of hair care products do not contain harmful ingredients, and they are also loaded with vitamins and minerals.

Use Products To Moisturize Your Hair

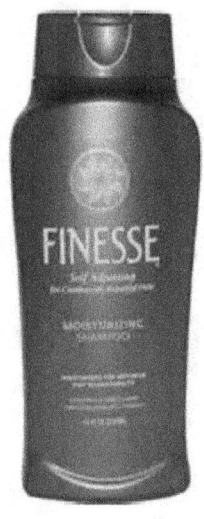

If you having problem with dry hair, it could become brittle easily, and that will hinder hair growth. You should make sure your hair moisturized at all times. You can keep your hair moisturized by using hair product, such as shampoos and conditioners.

Conditioning Your Hair

To be sure your hair is properly conditioned, if you are styling it often or not, you need to apply a leave in conditioner regularly. Doing this will make your hair healthier, and will also protect it from harsh elements.

Choose a hair conditioner that is made by a reputable company to ensure its quality.

Trim Your Hair Regularly

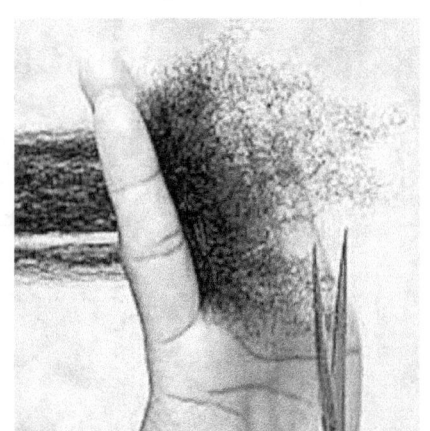

You may think this doesn't help your hair grow, but it can really help in speeding up its growth.

To trim your hair means that you cut only about a quarter to a half of an inch of your hair every six weeks. This will prevent your hair from becoming dry and dull, as well as prevent split ends, which all shorten its growth.

Protect Your Hair

You must understand that the tips of your hair are the oldest part of it. This means the tips are the areas that dry out first, causing split ends. You should make sure that the tips are protected from elements that can harm your hair.

Protect your hair from too much exposure to the sun. Exposure to sun for long periods will remove the healthy oils of your scape that help hair growth.

Protect Your Hair At Bedtime

It's very important that you always protect your hair at bedtime. This is because it is possible that you are rubbing your hair against a pillowcase, which can risk pulling hair out when you are sleeping. To stop this from happening, you should cover your hair, or make sure that you have a silk or satin pillowcase. These types of covers will prevent you from losing hair like you would on a cotton pillowcase.

You can also protect your hair by covering it with a hair net.

Did you know that massaging your scalp twice a day on a regular basis will help you achieve faster hair growth? This is because it actually stimulates your hair follicles.

It works best if your massage your hair when applying conditioner, or before brushing or styling it, so that it can look more sexy.

Dandruff Harms Your Hair Growth

Dandruff can stop your hair growth if it gets out of control because it is caused by a certain type of fungus that feeds on the oil of your scalp. You'll need to follow a hair care treatment that can prevent dandruff.

If you have dandruff, purchase a shampoo that can get rid of it as soon as you can.

Use Prenatal Supplements

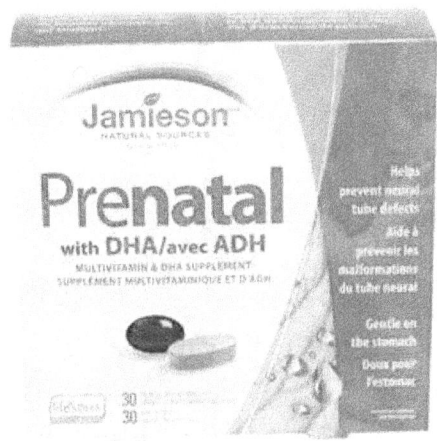

Have you ever wondered why pregnant women's hair grows so fast? This is because prenatal supplements, these types of supplements actually contain nutrients that contribute to hair growth. So, if you really want to grow hair faster, then I would start using these supplements today.

Grape Seed Oil

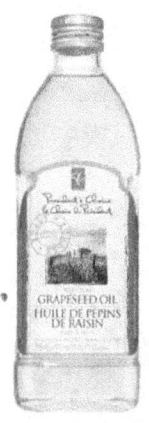

Using grape seed oil on your hair can result in faster hair growth in a few weeks. You need to apply it whenever you are massaging your scalp. For the best results, apply the oil just before you go to bed, this ensure that your scalp can absorb it to the fullest.

Most grocery stores carry grape seed oil. You'll find it in the pharmacy or health food area.

Cactus Leaves

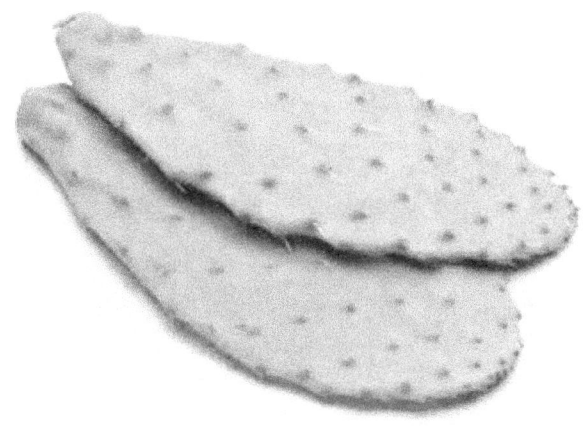

Cut out a few cactus leaves from a plant, and cut it into small pieces in a small pan of water and leave it overnight. The next morning, apply the water to your hair and leave it on for 1 hour. This treatment can make your hair grow fast, because cactus leaves adds many of its essential nutrients to the water when it soaks overnight.

Garlic, Onions, and Cinnamon Sticks

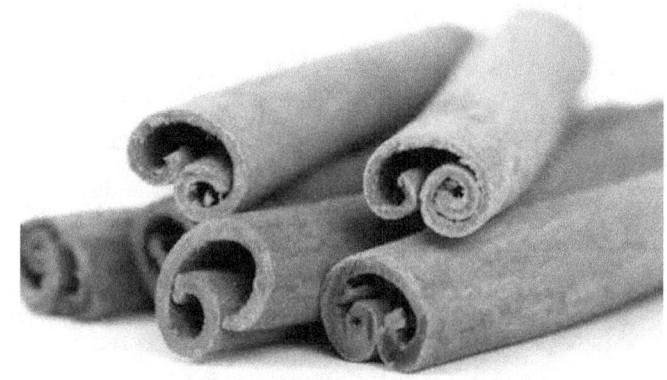

Step One: Mix two cinnamon sticks, four cloves of garlic, and a red onion

Step Two: Boil the mixture for 20 minutes, and let it cool down for 20 minutes.

Step Three: Apply it to your scalp and rinse after 1 hour. Use this treatment for a period of four consecutive days for maximum results.

Birth Control Pills and Your Shampoo

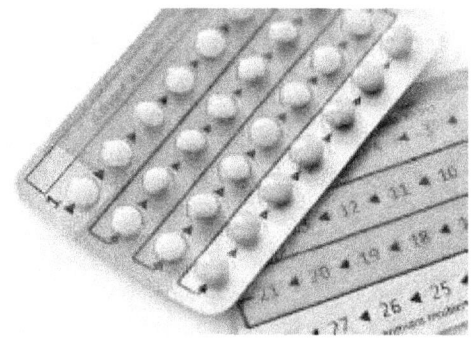

Birth control pills contain chemicals that can actually make your hair grow faster.

To use this treatment, grind five birth control pills into a powder and mix it into your bottle of shampoo.

Use your shampoo regularly, to see results in just a few weeks.

Thank you so much for taking the time to read this book. I hope your hair care regimen is an easy and simple process.

Now I'd like ask for a *small* favor. If you found this book to be useful, please take a few minutes to leave a review on Amazon...

...Even a few sentences will help!

Here's the link again:

amazon.com/author/marciasavage e

This feedback will help me to write the kind of Kindle books that help you get results. And if you loved it, please let me know.

Your Free Gift

As a way of saying thanks for your purchase, I'm offering a free guide that's exclusive to my readers.

In this guide, you will learn how to turn any messy room in into a nice, clean, and tidy room, cleaning in only 3 hours. Your home will stay clean every day and you will never have to worry about unexpected guests walking into a dirty house again. You can download this free report by going here.

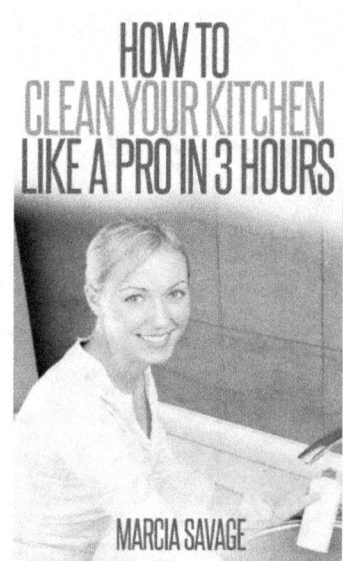

http://forms.aweber.com/form/76/315836976.htm

More Kindle eBooks By Marcia Savage:

CLEAN HOUSE IN 30 MINUTES

http://www.amazon.com/dp/B00HVS4TZG

NATURAL SKINCARE REMEDIES REVEAL

http://www.amazon.com/dp/B00J9OVE12

AN ORGANIZED HOME IN 30 MINUTES

http://www.amazon.com/dp/B00IHRCQHI

BEST HOMEMADE STAIN REMOVER EVER

http://www.amazon.com/dp/B00IPQ1VF4

Radiant Skin the Natural Way

http://www.amazon.com/dp/B00JAQWNFA

Kindle eBooks By Bernard Savage

At Last, A Proven Way To Housebreak Your Dog

http://www.amazon.com/dp/B00G

At Last, A Proven Way To Train A Well-Behaved Dog

http://www.amazon.com/dp/B00GWBEUYS

The Easy Way To Housebreak Your Dog In 10 Days

http://www.amazon.com/dp/B00HK9BIGE

The Easy Way To Teach Your Dog To Come In 10 Days

http://www.amazon.com/dp/B00HL24R40

The Easy Way To Train A Well-Behaved Dog In 10 Days

http://www.amazon.com/dp/B00HKUTB3A

GUARANTEED PROVEN RESULTS! TEACH YOUR DOG TO COME WHEN YOU CALL IN 10 DAYS

http://www.amazon.com/dp/B00H5CE3Y0

The Absolute Quickest Way To Start A Window Cleaning Business

http://www.amazon.com/dp/B00G

The Absolute Cheapest Way To Start A Doggy Daycare Business

http://www.amazon.com/dp/B00GKPDWFO

The Fastest Way To Start A Successful Pet Grooming Business

http://www.amazon.com/dp/B00GISLRQY

The Fast Way To Start A Car Detailing Business

http://www.amazon.com/dp/B00GH565ME

www.ingramcontent.com/pod-product-compliance
Lightning Source LLC
Chambersburg PA
CBHW080343290526
45791CB00009BA/2716